Natural Childbirth ~ How I Achieved Short Labors Without Drugs

by Monette Powell

Disclaimer:

Although this book covers health related topics, the information in this book is not intended to be a substitute for treatment or advice by a professional health care provider. The author and publisher are not responsible for any adverse consequences sustained by any person using the information in this book.

I am not a medical professional or nutritionist and this book is not medical advice. I was under the care of a medical doctor or midwife for each of my pregnancies and I discussed the things I share in this book with them and sought their advice and approval. The information I share is my own personal story and experience. There is no guarantee you would experience the same results.

Table of Contents

1. Introduction

My first childbirth experience was induced and a very painful one. Because of this, for many years I was afraid to have any more children. This is the story of my first childbirth experience and how I went on to have three more children, all without drugs and all with 3 1/2 to 4 hour labors that turned out to be great birth experiences!

The things I share in this book are from my own experiences with the pregnancies and births of my four children, what I have learned and what has worked for me personally. What I share is not meant to be medical advice. My hope is that what I share will be a help to someone else.

2. Benefits of Natural Childbirth

When I say natural childbirth, personally, it means to me that I had my babies while I was under the care of a doctor or midwife and my births were without the use of any drugs or medical interventions like cesarean births or episiotomies for example.

The benefits I experienced in childbirth without drugs are:

For me:
Increased energy, strength and alertness of mind during labor and after

Feeling in control of my body and birth experience

Freedom to move around without things attached to me like monitors and IV's

Minimal pain

Short labors

Having the energy after the birth to be
able to get up out of bed move
around freely and rather quickly

Quick recovery time

I could bond with my babies right away

No side effects from drugs

Financially it was cheaper than paying
for all the medical interventions

For my Babies:

They were alert and looking around right
after birth

They wanted to breastfeed right away

They had energy

They could make eye contact with me and weren't sleepy

Healthier because they were not subjected to the drugs and their side effects

3. My First Experience Giving Birth

I was married a month and a half after my 19th birthday. I look at my youngest daughter who just turned 18, almost the age that I was when I got married, and although she is mature for her age, like I was at that age, I ask myself, what in the world was I thinking? Why didn't my parents stop me?

Many people thought I was getting married because I was pregnant. I was asked that question many times. I suppose they thought that because of my young age, but it wasn't the reason.

I don't advise anyone to get married at such a young age. I know now that while I thought I was mature at that age, I still lacked knowledge of what life was really about. I didn't have time to experience life as a single person and I spent a lot of time regretting my decision.

I didn't really know myself well at that age to really know what I really needed in someone. It wasn't until I got into my late twenties to middle thirties that I really started to figure out what qualities I really needed in a spouse. So, I don't recommend getting married at a young age.

I was 22 when I had my first child. When my husband and I decided to have a baby, we tried for several months to conceive, but it did not happen. Not at first anyway.

I remember I was so focused on it that is all I could think about. I think because I was so focused on this, that maybe I was actually working against myself. I started to wonder if my body was capable of making a child or if there was something wrong with me.

I finally decided to just let it go, and if it happened, wonderful, and if not, I would be okay with that too. So, it was when I let it go and stopped worrying and thinking about it that it happened. I was finally pregnant! I was so excited and so happy that I would finally get to be a mom!

We had three house cats at the time and I remember the doctor telling me that I should not change the litter box while I was pregnant. I was happy to get out of this chore and have a reason for my husband to do it. The reason the doctor told me this was because of a parasitic infection that could possibly be transmitted to me through infected cat feces called Toxoplasmosis which could cause some serious birth defects in the baby. So, I was happy to turn over that job and have a break from it.

At this time of my life, I was a meat eater and didn't eat as healthy as I could have.

I was eating the best I knew how at that point in my life. I do remember eating lots of oranges and pineapple during my first pregnancy. I craved those. I also remember loving to drink cow milk and lots of it. Between my husband and I, we went through 5 gallons of milk a week. That was a lot of milk!

My favorite food was Mexican food at that time. When I got pregnant, I could no longer eat it. The thought of it made me feel sick. Even once I had my baby it was a whole year before I could eat Mexican food again. But it would never be my favorite food again. I rarely could eat it. To this day, I only have it on rare occasions. I don't know why, but something changed in me regarding that with that pregnancy.

I did start craving potatoes, and to this day, potatoes are one of my favorite foods. If I don't eat them after a few days, I still get cravings for them. They must contain something my body needs. This is the only food craving I get on a regular basis. Maybe it's just that I love potatoes.

During my whole pregnancy we were so sure we were going to have a boy that we only had a boy's name picked out. It was Matthew. We did not have a girl's name picked out at all.

I don't know about you, but when I was not pregnant, I could think of all these names, both of boys and girls names that I liked. When I was pregnant and it actually came down to picking one, I always had a hard time deciding on one.

I always struggled with the thought that whatever name I picked, this baby would have to live with it the rest of their life. Since I was made fun of in school as a kid, I wanted a name that people couldn't easily make fun of. Maybe silly, but that is the way I thought.

I was close to eight months pregnant when I joined a Lamaze class. On the night of the second class they took us to the hospital and gave us a tour of the maternity ward and delivery room and explained to us the process that we would go through when it was time to give birth. I found it all very informative and interesting. The reality hit me too, that it was getting close for me. I would soon be a mom, sooner than I realized.

I went home that night really feeling like I needed to come up with a name for a girl in case our baby was not going to be a boy. So, after doing some searching we came up with the name of Stephanie. It was the only name we could decide on that we both liked.

During this pregnancy I was working a full time job and the next day, I went to work as usual. I also had a routine doctor's appointment this day. While I was at the doctor he asked me what my plans were for the rest of the day. I told him that I was going to go back to work. He then informed me that I would not be doing that and that he was admitting me to the hospital instead. It really took me by surprise.

Even though I felt fine, it turns out I had something called Preeclampsia. My blood pressure was too high. Because of this I was going to be admitted to the hospital and my labor was going to be induced. I don't think he told me that at the office. He said I was going in for some bed rest. It wasn't until after I was admitted to the hospital that I was told I was going to have my labor induced.

I never did an ultrasound during my pregnancy because I did not want to know the sex of my baby. I wanted it to be a surprise. When I was admitted to the hospital they did do an ultrasound, but I told them I still did not want to know the sex of my baby.

I was taken to a labor room and hooked up to a monitor that went around my belly to monitor the baby's heartbeat. They started me on an IV, of who knows what. They also had me hooked up to a blood pressure machine with a cuff around my arm that would automatically take my blood pressure every 15 minutes. So, every 15 minutes my arm was being squeezed. They also gave me an enema. And I was made to stay on my back. Needless to say, I was very uncomfortable.

I would say they started to induce my labor around 5 or 6 pm. When they started running the drugs through the IV that would do this, it made my whole body feel like it was on fire. I remember feeling this burning sensation through my whole body which made me feel even worse.

I was so thirsty and had cotton mouth, yet they wouldn't let me have anything to drink. My blood pressure was high and the one thing I needed for that was water and they wouldn't let me have any. They would give me these cotton swabs to dip in water to rub inside my mouth. When the nurse left, I had my husband feeding me ice chips. I couldn't quit eating them I was so thirsty.

At one point, the nurse came in the room and saw him giving me the ice chips and she told him to stop doing that because I would throw up. When she left I told my husband that I wasn't going to throw up and please keep giving me the ice chips, which he did.

As the hours progressed, I started feeling more and more painful contractions brought on by the drugs they were giving me. I spent all this time on my back still hooked up to all these things which left me with little options to move around in any different positions to get comfortable.

By around 3 am, it was extremely painful and I wanted something for the pain. It was so bad, I think I was yelling at this point and I just kept saying over and over, "God help me get through this night!"

My husband was trying to calm me down by telling me to breathe how they told us to in the Lamaze class and I remember shouting at him, "Shut up and you breathe, I will breathe how I want to!"

Before they would give me anything for the pain, they came in with all this paperwork they wanted me to read regarding the dangers and wanted me to sign something releasing them from any consequences for any spinal injury.

I was in no state of mind to read anything or sign anything because I was in so much pain, so my husband had to do it. They gave me an epidural but I can say, it did not work on me. I still felt the pain just as much as ever.

My baby was about ready to be born and they moved me to a delivery room for the birth to happen. The same room I just saw the night before on the tour for my Lamaze class. I never would have guessed that night that I would be there the very next night going through this.

I remember them giving me an episiotomy (a surgical cut they make between the vagina and the anus to expand the opening of the vagina to prevent tearing during delivery). I did not feel this because of the epidural and all the other pain of the labor.

It was during these last few hours before my baby was born that I asked my doctor what he thought the baby was. He then told me he thought I was going to have a girl. I had just picked out her name the night before and I had just taken a tour of this hospital birthing area the night before and was told what the procedures would be. I was glad I had the tour so I would at least know what to expect. What timing!

My baby girl was born around 6:25 am. I remember hearing her cry for the first time and feeling relief from all the pain. They brought her up to my face to show her to me. I was so weak I couldn't even lift my head off of the pillow.

The doctor gave me stitches where the episiotomy was and stuck an ice pack between my legs. They tried to rush me out of the delivery room because they said they had another mother they needed to use the room for.

They brought a bed and wanted me to move over to it, but I had no energy to move. I remember it took two people to pick me up to move me to this new bed so they could wheel me out of the delivery room. They took me back to the same room where I spent the night laboring. After spending a few hours there they finally took me to a regular hospital room.

It was in this hospital room that I got to hold my baby for the first time and try to nurse her. It was a new joy I never experienced and such a neat feeling to hold this little person in my arms for the first time.

Once all the drugs wore off, I was starting to feel the pain of my stitches. I remember feeling like I didn't want to go to the bathroom. They also did not want me to get out of bed at first so they inserted a catheter.

I also found out later the doctor was considering doing a cesarean on me even though my baby's head was down and in the right position. My husband talked him out of it he said. I was so thankful.

They did release us from the hospital a few days later, but our baby had to be readmitted to the hospital because she had jaundice and her bilirubin was too high. So, we had to spend more time in the hospital until this could be brought down. I don't remember how long we had to be there but she had to stay in an incubator with lights on her. They said she was about 5 weeks early.

They eventually released us from the hospital and then she had to be in an incubator in our house and still had to stay under the lights for what seemed like a couple more weeks. This was an ordeal.

We had to have a nurse come to the house to check on her every day, but after a period of time, she could finally be out of this for good, and that was a big relief.

It was very stressful going through this as a new mom. I did not get much rest. You want everything to go smoothly and be ok and you worry about whether your baby will be okay.

They were talking at one point of the possibility of giving her a blood transfusion which we did not want to do. Thankfully, she never had to have that.

4. Getting Healthy Before Getting Pregnant

After my first experience, I was so scared of ever having another baby. I did not want to go through what I did the first time. It was so painful and I did not want to go through that pain again. So, I was not planning on ever having any more kids, ever!

It was after my first baby was born that I would go to the grocery store and I remember going to the meat section and looking at all those dead animal parts laying there and hating to have to buy it.

I remember wishing I knew how to be a vegetarian, but didn't know the first thing about it. It was a desire in my heart to be one, but I didn't know anyone who was one or how to begin.

For the next two years, we still ate the meat and the dairy and nothing in our diet changed. For the first two years of my daughter's life she was always having ear infections and upper respiratory infections. I was always taking her to the doctor for one of these problems and they would prescribe the usual drugs for those things but they would never work.

It was when she was about two that I came across a book called _Counsels on Diet and Foods_ by Ellen G. White. This book forever changed the course of my life regarding diet and lifestyle and led me down a path to start doing my own research on healthy topics and make healthy changes in my diet and lifestyle.

I read this book from cover to cover. It had been exactly what I was looking for. It was the information I needed on how to become a vegetarian, so I ate it up.

I was never a coffee drinker, but I loved to drink Lipton iced tea and Dr. Pepper. I never thought I was addicted to caffeine, but when I tried to give up the Lipton iced tea and the Dr. Pepper; I did experience withdrawal symptoms and headaches which let me know I was addicted to the caffeine after all.

We got off all meat, dairy, sugar and white flour products and I started substituting them with wholesome foods. I started using food in its natural state as much as possible and cooking from scratch, not using processed prepackaged foods.

I was not fat but when I did change my diet to be healthier, I did lose weight and when I stopped eating meat, I remember feeling like this big weight was taken off my body.

I started having salads and eating fresh fruit, using whole grains (like brown rice instead of white rice for example), beans and nuts. I started learning how to make cheese from cashews. I started baking my own bread.

I found some good vegan cookbooks and started teaching myself how to prepare food this way without meat and dairy. And at least for me, I found it more interesting with more variety, and more rewarding and fun to eat healthfully than the way I was eating before. The way I was eating before, I actually dreaded cooking anything.

Remember when I said I never thought I would ever give up milk? Well, I never thought it possible, but I did and it's been almost thirty years now since I have. I have no regrets about that decision and haven't looked back. Now, I use almond or coconut milk most often, and sometimes cashew milk too. You can find some pretty good ones out there or make your own, which I have done also.

I made all the changes to our diet that I was reading about within three months and we became a vegan family. I can say that once I did this, my daughter no longer had any more ear infections or upper respiratory infections. In fact, I didn't have to make any more trips to the doctor because she didn't get sick any more.

I continued to study more and more on my own about natural health. I started reading herb books, juicing books, vegetarian cook books and all kinds of natural health books.

I had always been a city girl, and was used to everything being so convenient and having stores just down the street. I never thought I could live in the country.

We had an opportunity to move on a big ranch out in the country. A friend was able to get a nice house on this ranch for us to rent. At first, I was scared to death of moving to the country. I thought I would see a rattlesnake behind every rock. But, it wasn't the case. I know they are out there, but I never ran across any.

I was afraid of spiders and bugs. I did have to encounter these, and did have to learn how to kill them. I remember the first time I encountered a scorpion in my sink. I about had a heart attack, literally.

I didn't know how to kill one, and was afraid that if I tried to smash it with something it would jump at me. My heart was pounding from fear as I was trying to figure out what to do to kill it. First I tried to pour some Listerine mouth wash on it. This just made it run around the sink. Next, I tried to pour some Clorox on it, and it did the same thing. Finally, I just decided to try to smash it. So, I grabbed the Listerine bottle and smashed it with that. It seemed to work, but I had to do it several more times to make sure it was dead.

After that, I was always on the lookout for the scorpions that would come up the drain. I remember I prayed every day that I would never get stung. I never did, even though one day I had opened up a dish cloth that was folded in the kitchen sink and when I did, out ran a scorpion onto my wrist. I flung the washcloth and scorpion across the room. Another time, I had picked up a big book and set it on my lap and there was a scorpion on the edge of the outside pages. Thankfully, I didn't get stung then either.

I used to have dreams at night that they were crawling all over my bed, but that wasn't the case, even though they will get in your bed. Living in the country does take some getting used to, but it is a huge blessing in many ways. I have always lived in the country since then and love it. You learn to deal with the critters, especially living in Texas, which is where I was at the time. And that is the best place to learn to get used to them, for Texas has lots of them.

5. Baby Number Two

There is a six year and eight month difference between my first child and my second child. It took me a long time to get up the nerve to try for another child. For the longest time, I just thought I would like to adopt. I did not want to go through another painful delivery like the first one I had. I started having a strong desire in my heart to have another baby.

I had spent the years between my first child and second child doing a lot of studying on natural health subjects, changing my diet to a vegan diet and learning about eating healthy. I did much reading about the benefits of using herbs instead of drugs and learning about juicing and the different benefits of different juices, etc.

By the time I was pregnant with my second child, I had learned a lot that I didn't know when I was pregnant the first time. My diet was totally different now, and I was living a much healthier lifestyle, a totally different lifestyle than I did during my first pregnancy. Even my surroundings were different. I was more in the country than the city.

By the time I was pregnant with my second child, we had moved to a different town that was nearly three hours away from where I was when I had my first baby.

In this new location I came in contact with people that home schooled their children. I also had a desire to do this before I moved but didn't know anyone who did this. So, I was happy to meet some people who were already doing it.

I started learning all I could from them, and many of them too, lived healthy lifestyles, so I found some people I could learn from both in home schooling and vegetarianism.

I was pregnant with my second child and I desired to not use drugs at all in this pregnancy. I wanted to apply the things I had learned and do things differently this time. I needed to find a doctor who would work with me on this. I really desired to have a midwife and have a baby at home, but my husband wouldn't let me. He was too worried something would go wrong considering my first experience.

So, I started asking some of the homeschoolers I knew if they could recommend a good doctor that was also into natural childbirth and would not push the drugs but let me have a baby naturally. Several people recommended this one certain doctor to me, so I got several good reviews about her.

I had been to two men gynecologists in my life and felt like they were not very sensitive to my needs and then I started questioning whether I should even be going to a man doctor for female issues. Somewhere along the line, I decided I wanted to use a woman from now on.

So, I went to visit this woman doctor. She was actually a family practice doctor who also delivered babies. She was very friendly and I liked her right from the beginning. She was also very much into natural childbirth. At the time I knew her, she had six kids of her own and she had given birth to them all at home. So, she definitely believed in natural childbirth and home births.

I chose to go with her. It was really important to me that I find a health care provider that shared my same beliefs and that would work with me on the kind of childbirth experience I wanted to have. While she didn't deliver babies at home, she did let you have a natural experience in the hospital. Since my husband didn't want me to have a home birth, this was a great option for me.

I want to say here, that everything I did, I talked over with my doctor and later my midwife first to know if it was ok for me to do.

During my first pregnancy, I used prenatal vitamins that the doctor prescribed, but they also constipated me.

I did not want to use prenatal vitamins again, so I didn't. What I did instead, was ate a very healthful vegan diet which included fresh fruit, salads, whole grains, beans, nuts, and I was also juicing carrots with a combination of celery, beets, and spinach. I did this for baby number two, three and four. I have four kids altogether.

Since I had read so much about herbs over the last few years, I learned about Red Raspberry leaf tea. Some of the benefits are that it increases fertility, strengthens the uterus to help prepare for childbirth and helps reduce the pain in childbirth.

It is full of many nutrients like A, B complex, iron, calcium, phosphorus, potassium and magnesium to name a few.   It is also helpful in reducing morning sickness. I highly suggest you go read further about this wonderful herb. It is good for so many female issues and pregnancy.

Just a side note (fast forward to present), I was having an issue within the last year regarding my periods lasting too long and being too heavy (going through some premenopausal changes). I have always been regular with my periods all my life and so this was out of the ordinary for me. I was doing some reading on Red Raspberry leaf tea again, and was reminded of its benefits and even of its benefits for this stage of life also. It helps reduce menstrual cramps (which I have never had, thankfully) and helps regulate the flow of menstruation and decreases heavy periods. So, I drank some and even after one cup of it, my flow was reduced to just spotting within a couple of hours.

I used the loose leaf Red Raspberry tea during my pregnancies, but if you can't find that, use the tea bags. Organic is always best. Each morning during my pregnancy, I would make a quart of the tea that I would drink throughout the day. I started this early in my pregnancy. I would not put any sweetener in it.

Somewhere I read or heard that if you used sweetener in an herbal tea when you are trying to use it for medicinal purposes it would neutralize the effect you are trying to accomplish. I don't know if that is true or not, but I did not put any sweetener in it just in case. It does not taste bad to me plain.

My pregnancy with baby two went really well. I did not experience any problems or complications. With all my pregnancies, I never even had any morning sickness, which was a blessing. I read the Raspberry Leaf tea is good for helping with relieving morning sickness if you do have some.

When I got to the last 5-6 weeks of my pregnancy, I used an herbal combination by Nature's Sunshine called 5-W. It is an herbal combination that you specifically take during the last 5-6 weeks of your pregnancy to help with the birth. I followed the directions on the bottle for taking this supplement.

With my second baby my labor started around midnight. I never knew with any of my pregnancies after the first one, whether I was really in labor or not because the pain was mild. I was hesitant about going to the hospital because I didn't want it to just be a false alarm and not the real thing. I did go with this one just to be sure, and sure enough, it was the real thing.

My husband took me to the hospital, and my dear sweet mother went with me. She was always so sweet to stay with me to help me before and after each baby was born. Even my daughter who was close to seven went also. My doctor allowed them all to be in the room during the birth.

I was completely alert, and I was surprised that I had so much energy compared to my first experience. The pain was minimal and bearable and not really that bad. The only time it got worse was the last fifteen minutes before the baby was born. And that was mainly because of the strong urge to push. I only had to push maybe ten minutes with this baby and he, yes a boy, was out. This labor lasted about four hours from the time I started feeling contractions until he was actually out.

This birth was so much better than the first one. I did not use any drugs. The pain was much less and it was bearable. The doctor did not do an episiotomy. I did tear just a little where she had to give me one or two stitches, but the pain of that was much less and the healing time much faster.

In my first labor, they would not let me drink anything. In this labor, my second one, I was allowed to have my quart bottle of water and drink as much as I wanted. After this baby was born, they did give me some apple juice because I developed a headache.

So, in my next two births, I had my quart of water and my quart of apple juice by my bed which I drank during the labor and after. No one ever tried to take it away or tell me I couldn't have it because

I was going to throw up. In fact, the issue was never even brought up by any of the medical staff.

They only hooked me up to a monitor when I first arrived to get the heartbeat of the baby then they took it off and it stayed off. I had no IV's and nothing attached to me.

My new son was so alert. I remember him looking at me and looking around the room. He also nursed right away.

I was able to get up out of bed within the hour and go to the bathroom and take a shower. I did not feel tired like I did with the first one when I was all drugged up. I had energy and so did my baby.

I was also able to keep my baby in my room the majority of the time instead of the nursery.

I spent a day and a half in the hospital. The only reason it was the extra half day was because we were waiting on the doctor to come release us.

My first and second labors were night and day experiences. They were so different from each other. I was glad that I decided to have another child.
This experience went so well, I was no longer afraid to have another…

6. Baby Number Three

My first two babies were planned. I had purposely tried to get pregnant. My third baby was a surprise. I was not trying to get pregnant, but it happened. And I knew the day it happened, and just knew in my heart I was going to be pregnant, and sure enough I was.

I had a struggle with this one in the sense that I was not mentally prepared for another child. With the first two, I had planned it, and was mentally prepared, had time to think about it. This one was unexpected and it kind of threw me into a little stressful feeling mode of not feeling ready. I felt overwhelmed with the thought of a third child.

I did the same things as I did with my second pregnancy. I used the same doctor I did with my second child. I ate a healthy vegan diet and did the juicing instead of the prenatal vitamins, took the

Red Raspberry tea throughout my pregnancy and used the herbal combination 5-W the last 5-6 weeks of my pregnancy.

My labor started around 11:30 to midnight, and again, I wasn't sure if it was the real thing or not. I waited a bit longer than I should have to go to the hospital with this one. I was really not sure if I was in labor.

We decided to go to the hospital. I remember walking out to the car and I had this urge to go to the bathroom, so I went back up to the front door of our house to go in to use the bathroom. When I got to the door and was about to go inside, I had another contraction. I decided that I better not take the time to go to the bathroom, so I got into the car so we could be on our way.

My contractions were becoming stronger and my husband was trying to hurry. We came upon some railroad tracks where the gates had come down and the lights were flashing because a train was coming.

My husband decided not to wait for the train to pass so he drove around the gates and crossed the tracks. He sped to the hospital and by the time we got there my contractions were much stronger and closer together.

They admitted me right away and when they wheeled me to my room in the wheel chair, they took me to the exact same room I had been about two years prior, the same room I was in when I had my second baby. I felt like I was reliving the same experience. My water broke after they got me to the room and into the bed.

This was a very fast delivery. The doctor did not make it to the hospital in time to deliver this baby because I had him about twenty minutes after I arrived there. The nurse delivered this baby and the doctor arrived in time to deliver the afterbirth.

It was a good thing we did not wait for that train or I feel certain that I would have had my baby in the car. And it was a good thing I decided to get in the car instead of taking the time to go to the bathroom or we would not have been able to go around the gates at the railroad tracks.

This baby's birth was much like the last one, about four hours and the pain was bearable. I remember just giving a few pushes and he was out. Yes, another boy. This third baby we named Matthew, the name we originally thought we would name our first child that we thought was going to be a boy.

I remember lying in bed after this baby's birth and hearing a woman in the next room screaming her head off trying to give birth. I felt sorry for her and wished that I could have helped ease her pain some. I was very thankful mine was over with and that I did not have the pain she apparently was having.

This baby was also very alert and was looking around right after being born. He also started nursing right away. I felt energetic and was able to be up within the hour of delivering him. I did not tear with this baby and did not need any stitches.

Another great experience….

7. Using a Midwife for Baby Number Four

After I had my third baby, I constantly had this feeling that someone was missing, and was always looking around for a fourth kid because it just felt like another one should be there. This feeling went on continuously, until I got pregnant with my next baby.

By the time I was pregnant with my fourth child and I went back to see my doctor, she had decided to stop delivering babies so I was not able to use her for my fourth baby.

I really wanted to have a home birth, and it had been what I wanted all along. I could not find another doctor like her, so this time my husband was okay with my getting a midwife for this pregnancy since my other two went so well.

Again, I asked people I knew if they could refer me to any good midwives. I visited with three different ones before deciding on one I liked.

The one I chose fit well with my personality and she seemed kind and gentle and shared many of my same beliefs.

Another thing I really liked about her was the fact that I never had to leave my house for any of my visits with her. She always came to see me for my visits and she did the blood draws at my home. I really loved the conveniences of her services. I always felt kind of stressed out having to go sit in a doctor's waiting room.

Her price was much more reasonable too than other midwives that I talked to who expected me to drive to them for my monthly visits.

The midwife I chose only charged us 1200.00 for the whole birth and all of her services including my monthly in home visits. A real bargain compared to any hospital birth.

I really loved the fact that I knew I would not be leaving my home for anything, visits or going to any hospital. All this made me feel more relaxed to know I could stay in the comfort of my own home.

With my two boy babies, I did have ultra sounds to find out what their sex was. So, I knew they were boys before they were born. With this baby, since I wasn't going to any hospitals I did not have an ultrasound and this baby remained a mystery as to what it would be, same as my first one.

My midwife suspected this baby was going to be a girl. She was right. There are certain ways they can determine what it might be, at least this lady could, without having an ultrasound.

One of the ways she told me she could tell was because I had problems early on with having a vaginal yeast infection. I've never had any yeast infections in my life. Only when I was pregnant did I have them, but they were usually only the last month or so. She told me that girl babies produce more hormones.

I was taking my Raspberry tea daily again and doing the juicing, eating a healthy vegan diet. Again, I used the 5-W herbal combination at the end of this pregnancy as well.

I was also using another product at this time called Herbal Fiberblend. It is a product that helps you stay regular and will also help kill parasites and their eggs inside your intestines. It contains herbs that help to cleanse your body of toxins.

It does have a note on the container that if you are pregnant or nursing you should consult a health practitioner before using this. My midwife told me since I was using this product before I was pregnant, that it would be ok to continue it during my pregnancy. So, I did.

I was also drinking barley grass juice, which I also continued to take during my pregnancy. Later, I will tell you how you can get these two great items and give you a list of the other items I mentioned.

When it was time for this baby to be born I was able to stay in bed this time and just relax at first. Again, I wasn't sure if I was really in labor, so I was even hesitant to call the midwife. I don't know why all my babies wanted to come during the night, but they did. The last three all started around 11:30 to midnight and were all born around 3:30 to 4 am. This baby was my shortest labor. She was about three and a half hours total from the time I felt the first contraction to the time she was born.

I started feeling my contractions, but I was able to stay in bed and half way sleep for a while. Then they became stronger and closer together. At this point it was uncomfortable for me to stay in bed. So I then got up and just walked around the house for the rest of the time. It was at this point that I decided to call the midwife. By then, my contractions were much closer together, I'd say like five minutes apart.

She arrived in time and she also brought an assistant to help her. Prior to this, she gave me a list of things to do and supplies to have on hand to be prepared for this birth.

I also had a waterbed at the time, but she said I couldn't have a baby on the waterbed. So we pulled the mattress out of our sofa in the living room and put it on the floor of the bedroom which would be for the new baby. We had this prepared ahead of time. We made the room all comfortable and had all the supplies in there the midwife told us to be prepared with.

I was up walking around the whole time until about maybe the last fifteen minutes before the birth of my daughter. I remember I had gone into the bathroom and as I was coming out I had to hold on to the entrance of the doorway for support because I was now having a strong urge to push all of a sudden.

It was at that point the midwife had me come into the bedroom and get on the mattress to prepare for the birth. I was having a hard time even walking to the bedroom to get on the mattress, because the contractions were so strong now, I just kept wanting to push.

As soon as I got situated on the mattress it was then that my water broke. I pushed maybe three times and she was born. The midwife was really great. She actually guided me when to push and how much while she rubbed oil on me to prevent me from tearing. She told me I had the clearest water she had ever seen.

Once my baby was out, she laid her up on my stomach right away face down and waited about fifteen minutes before she cut the cord. That was a whole new experience for me. None of the doctors ever did that. While she was lying on my stomach and she did pee on me. At that point you don't care, you need a shower anyway.

After the cord was cut, and the baby was checked out, weighed and measured, she then prepared a nice hot herbal bath for us. This was all new to me, but it was so nice. After I got in, she gave my daughter to me so I could hold her in the tub with me.

At this point my second child had awoke and he was always good even still to this day of coming up with just the funniest things to say at the right moment. He was about four years old at this time, and he came into the bathroom and saw us in the tub and the first thing he said was, "Mom, how come you are still fat?" He could see the baby was out, but my stomach still looked like she was in. I had to explain to him that it just doesn't instantly go back to its original size. After all, it took nine months to get to that size.

This was by far my best most relaxed experience. I am glad that I was able to experience all the deliveries I did even though the first one was the toughest. I realize it was because of all medical interventions that made the first one the hardest.

My last three births were the best and the last one was even better because it could be done at home in my own environment and in the comfort of familiar surroundings.

I could be up walking around or laying down in my own positions to make the labor go along smoothly and as comfortably as I could make it for myself instead of being made to stay in a bed in a certain position.

In the hospital, I think they train the babies to wake up at night. Don't ask me why they have to come into your room at odd hours of the night to wake the baby and you up.

One particular night with my third baby, we were all sleeping away, and at 1 am a nurse comes into our room, flips on all the lights, and announces it's time to give the baby a bath. What? At 1 am?

Seriously, what were they thinking? Couldn't that be done during the day?

When I had my baby at home, for the first two nights in a row, she slept through the whole night without waking up and it gave me some much needed rest also.

8. Simple Tips for Choosing a Health Care Provider

The following are some simple things you can do in searching for the right health care provider:

Do your research. Read about all the different kinds of birthing experiences there are. Read and learn from other women's experiences. I would talk to other women about their experiences.

Decide what kind of birth you want, whether it be in a hospital, birthing center or at home and what kind of health care provider you would like to use, whether it be an OB-GYN, Family Practice Doctor who delivers babies, or a Midwife for example.

Once you know what kind of birth experience you would like to have, ask people you know for recommendations or if they know of anyone who could recommend any good health care providers who would suit your needs.

Talk to others who have used any of the health care providers you may be considering or that have been recommended to you and find out what their experience was with that particular health care provider.

Make appointments with any health care providers you are considering and talk to them about your desires, concerns and the kind of birth experience you would like to have to find out if they can accommodate your requests and see if you feel comfortable using this person. Also, talk to them about any health concerns you may have.

9. Things I learned In My Own Experience

My first experience was with an OB-GYN Doctor. It was less personalized, and I felt like everything was done by the book or routine and there were many interventions. However, I did have a problem with my blood pressure, so at that time this was the best option for me. It was also all I knew about at that time.

I did get some recommendations from some people to use this doctor so I went with it. I also wonder though, had I been living a more healthy lifestyle and been on a better diet, would I have still had the same problem with my blood pressure? I did not have that problem in any of my last three pregnancies.

Once I got a little wiser and did more studying, I knew I didn't want to have the same experience I did the first time, so I started studying for myself other options and how I could make things better the next time. By the time I was ready to try to have another baby, I knew what kind of birth experience I wanted.

For my second and third babies, I used a Family Practice Doctor who also delivered babies and I had many good recommendations from different people who had good experiences with her. She was also in line with what I believed in and wanted and believed in home birth herself and practiced it in her own life.

She was a good option for me because she would work with me in having a natural child birth experience, yet in a hospital birth room setting in case there were complications. I felt I received more personal one on one care from her, and she wasn't so routine like the first doctor was. I was able to make more decisions and have things the way I wanted. There were no interventions in my two birth experiences with her.

And lastly, I was able to use a Midwife for my fourth child and have everything from the visits to the birth done from my home. I felt the midwife gave me the most personalized individual care and spent the most time with me. There were no other patients waiting outside the door in a waiting room. So, she had the time to give to me. She was more accessible by phone if I had any questions.

When it was time to deliver the baby, there were no interventions, and I was actually being coached when to push and how hard, to work with my body to facilitate a smooth delivery. The Midwife was also the least expensive.

Do your research and find the best options for your health situation and beliefs and find someone who will work with you on the kind of birth experience you want to have.

10. A Few More Healthy Tips

Get yourself healthy before you get pregnant! Study and read about what is the best diet for you. Diet makes a big difference in health. When I was growing up, I gave no thought to what I ate. Since I have done so much reading, I now see how important the relation to what we eat and how it affects our health really is.

Get some exercise every day. During my pregnancies, I walked.

After each pregnancy, it was harder for me to lose the weight, but once I started walking, the weight came off.

If I didn't have a very good place to walk or it was hard because I had other small children, where I couldn't just get up and go out when I wanted to, I did have my back yard. I went out in it twice a day and walked around it for twenty minutes two times a day. It made a difference.

You could also have a treadmill in your home if getting out is too difficult. I recently sold my elliptical machine to a lady who just had a baby. She was buying it to be able to lose weight after her pregnancy.

Get outside and get some fresh air and sunshine each day if you can.

I also prayed for my babies. I had many answered prayers for them and surrounding their births. For example, one thing I prayed for was that when I found out my second baby was going to be due in the same month I was born in, I prayed he would be born the day after my birthday, and he was! I prayed for many more things than this, but that is just one example.

11. Breastfeeding

Breastfeeding has many benefits for you and your baby. Breast milk contains antibodies that help your baby fight off sickness. It's just healthier, and the way God designed it.

With my first baby, it was hard at first to get her to start nursing right after birth. I know now it was because of all the drugs they gave me during labor. She was hard to wake up and wanted to sleep all the time. I struggled with nursing her and was tempted to give up. But, I am telling you, don't give up.

My nipples would get sore at first, but after a few weeks, they would toughen up and this wasn't a problem anymore. Usually, the first couple weeks are the hardest, but stick with it, it gets better.

Unfortunately, I went back to work full time with my first baby, so I gave up breast feeding her by the time she was three months. I really do regret that. I feel we missed important bonding time.

With the rest of my other babies, I was determined to not work even if I had to be poor. I wanted to be home with them. I nursed the boys for about two years and my last one until she was three.

I can't begin to tell you what a blessing it is to breastfeed your baby and get all that bonding time with them. After my third baby was weaned, I remember I wanted to have another baby so I could breast feed again. I can't explain it, but it gives a lot of satisfaction and joy.

I remember once I was pumping some breast milk one day and I was wondering what it tasted like. I decided to give it a try and tasted a little. I was really surprised to find out how sweet it was. It literally tasted like milk and honey. My reaction was, Wow, now I know why babies like it so much!

I would put my babies on a feeding schedule three hours apart but at the same times each day. This made them happier and less fussy and gave me some rest between feedings. It made it easier to get them to sleep through the night or most of the night by around six weeks.

For me, as long as I nursed my baby at least five times a day, it would keep my periods away. When I started to do less than five times a day as they got older, it would return. It was so nice to not have a period for about three years at a time between the pregnancy and nursing.

I also observed that the more raw foods I ate, like salads, fresh fruits and juices, the more milk I would have. If I ever felt like I was getting low on milk, I would go make some fresh carrot juice. I would then have so much milk my baby would be gulping it down.

I also noticed when I drank the barley juice and when I would pump, the milk would have a nice cream on top versus times when I wasn't using the barley juice.

So, I encourage you to breastfeed...and don't give up in discouragement. It's a great blessing for you and your baby in so many ways. You just have to experience it!

12. About My Kids And I

I've never been much of a career type person. My main desire in life was that I wanted to be a wife and a mom. This I have accomplished.

I have held jobs and I do now mainly out of the necessity to survive. It has never been my desire to climb some corporate ladder.

I hold no degrees, never went to college and only have a high school education with some extra classes I've taken here and there from time to time.

The majority of the jobs I have had have been in accounting. I have always had an interest in accounting and did take those types of classes in high school. I never had the money to go to college and refused to get into debt trying to go. So, I decided I would learn by getting jobs where I could get the experience instead and this is what I have done.

I absolutely love the job I have now working in accounting. But, even as much as I love the job I have now, I have to say though, the most rewarding job I ever had was the job of raising my kids.

It has brought me the most joys and satisfaction even though there were many frustrating times too. I look back and the best job and best years of my life were the eleven years I was a stay at home mom. Years I wish I could have back gladly.

Those years went by so quickly even though I thought it would be forever before my kids would be grown. Back then, I sometimes longed for the days when my kids would be grown and I could have some peace and quiet and time to myself. Now, I have lots of peace and quiet.

I remember I used to escape to the bathroom for five minutes of alone time only to have one or two of my kids knocking on the bathroom door wanting to come in, and the frustrating feeling I would have of not being able to be alone for five minutes! I would gladly take back those times today, for I miss them and being with my kids who have now started lives of their own.

If you are a new mom or about to become one, cherish those times with your kids and enjoy them as much as you can. Don't wish those years to go by, they will soon enough.

I have four beautiful healthy children who are now grown. My youngest just turned 18. My oldest is 29 and I am 51 at the time of this writing. I have two grandsons.

Two of my children are now married and two are not. My two sons are serving in the US Navy as did my father. My oldest daughter is married, and works for the US Postal Service, and she is the one who has two sons. My youngest just graduated from high school and is still living with me. We have a great relationship.

I have always had an interest in natural health subjects and became a vegan in 1988. I raised my children vegan. We were always healthy with nothing more than an occasional cold since we changed our diet.

I love exercise and do a lot of walking, running and hiking. My daughter and I also enjoy doing nature photography.

13. Some of My Favorite books, Supplements and Other Things

I would like to share just a few of my many favorite books that I have in my personal library that hopefully will be a blessing to you for further reading. You should be able to find these books on Amazon.

Counsels on Diet and foods ~ Ellen G. White (This is the book that changed the course of my life and started me down the path to changing my diet and lifestyle)

Ministry of Healing ~ Ellen G. White

Male Practice: How Doctors Manipulate Women ~ Robert S. Mendelsohn M.D.

How to Raise a Healthy Child in Spite of Your Doctor ~ Robert S. Mendelsohn M.D.

Confessions of a Medical Heretic ~ Robert S. Mendelsohn M.D.

A Shot in the Dark ~ H. Coulter

Natural Healing with Herbs: The Complete Reference Book for the Use of Herbs ~ Humbart Santillo

Nutritional Herbology: A Reference Guide to Herbs ~ Mark Pedersen

Fresh Vegetable and Fruit Juices ~ Dr. N. W. Walker D.Sc. and Dr. Norman W. Walker (This book is great and actually gives you juice combinations and measurements for different ailments)

Country Life Vegetarian Cookbook: Delicious Recipes from the Kitchens of the Country Life Vegetarian Restaurants ~ Diana Fleming

Forks over Knives ~ the Cookbook: Over 300 Recipes for Plant-Based Eating All through the Year

Nutritional Supplements:

Below are some of my favorite herbs and supplements I mentioned in this book that I used during my pregnancy and/or after:

Red Raspberry Leaf Tea, Organic (I used the Alvita brand during my pregnancies, but have also used the brand Traditional Medicinals, to help stop my bleeding for heavy menstrual flow in the last two years). You can get this at a health food store or on Amazon.

Nature's Sunshine 5-W Herbal Combination Supplement (I took this during the last 5-6 weeks of each of my last three pregnancies) I found it at health food stores. Amazon also sells it.

AIM Herbal Fiberblend is good for everyday use. Not necessary to have this just because you are pregnant. Get medical approval before you use this if you are pregnant or nursing.

AIM BarleyLife is the juice of young barley plants. You can order this and AIM Herbal Fiberblend at wholesale by going to this link:

http://myaimstore.com/aiming4health

Kitchen Appliances:

Some of my favorite things to use in the kitchen:

Champion Juicer (I have the commercial model)

Vitamix ~ Great to use as a blender and/or make some great soups and smoothies.

Kidalog Baby Food Mill Grinder ~ I used one like this with my kids. I did not buy baby food, except on rare occasions. I would use this baby food grinder to feed my toddlers and feed them what we were eating.

Oyama All Stainless Steel Rice Cooker ~ I love this rice cooker. The pot that the rice is cooked in is actually stainless steel.

Notes: